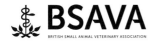
BSAVA
BRITISH SMALL ANIMAL VETERINARY ASSOCIATION

BSAVA Cognitive Aids for Anaesthesia
in Small Animal Practice

Matt McMillan
BVM&S DipECVAA AFHEA MRCVS
RCVS & European Recognised Specialist in Veterinary Anaesthesia
The Ralph Veterinary Referral Centre
Fourth Avenue, Globe Business Park
Marlow, Buckinghamshire SL7 1YG

T0200378

Published by:
British Small Animal Veterinary Association
Woodrow House, 1 Telford Way,
Waterwells Business Park, Quedgeley,
Gloucester GL2 2AB

A Company Limited by Guarantee in England
Registered Company No. 2837793
Registered as a Charity

A catalogue record for this book is available from the British Library.

ISBN 978 1 910443 75 0

The publishers, editors and contributors cannot take responsibility for
information provided on dosages and methods of application of drugs
mentioned or referred to in this publication. Details of this kind must be
verified in each case by individual users from up to date literature
published by the manufacturers or suppliers of those drugs. Veterinary
nurses are reminded that in each case they must follow all appropriate
national legislation and regulations from time to time in force.

Printed in the UK by Cambrian Printers Ltd, Pontllanfraith NP12 2YA
Printed on ECF paper made from sustainable forests
11314PUBS20

Titles in the BSAVA Manuals series:

Manual of Avian Practice: A Foundation Manual
Manual of Backyard Poultry Medicine and Surgery
Manual of Canine & Feline Abdominal Imaging
Manual of Canine & Feline Abdominal Surgery
Manual of Canine & Feline Advanced Veterinary Nursing
Manual of Canine & Feline Anaesthesia and Analgesia
Manual of Canine & Feline Behavioural Medicine
Manual of Canine & Feline Cardiorespiratory Medicine
Manual of Canine & Feline Clinical Pathology
Manual of Canine & Feline Dentistry and Oral Surgery
Manual of Canine & Feline Dermatology
Manual of Canine & Feline Emergency and Critical Care
Manual of Canine & Feline Endocrinology
Manual of Canine & Feline Endoscopy and Endosurgery
Manual of Canine & Feline Fracture Repair and Management
Manual of Canine & Feline Gastroenterology
Manual of Canine & Feline Haematology and Transfusion Medicine
Manual of Canine & Feline Head, Neck and Thoracic Surgery
Manual of Canine & Feline Musculoskeletal Disorders
Manual of Canine & Feline Musculoskeletal Imaging
Manual of Canine & Feline Nephrology and Urology
Manual of Canine & Feline Neurology
Manual of Canine & Feline Oncology
Manual of Canine & Feline Ophthalmology
*Manual of Canine & Feline Radiography and Radiology:
    A Foundation Manual*
*Manual of Canine & Feline Rehabilitation, Supportive and Palliative Care:
    Case Studies in Patient Management*
Manual of Canine & Feline Reproduction and Neonatology
*Manual of Canine & Feline Shelter Medicine: Principles of Health and
    Welfare in a Multi-animal Environment*
Manual of Canine & Feline Surgical Principles: A Foundation Manual
Manual of Canine & Feline Thoracic Imaging
Manual of Canine & Feline Ultrasonography
Manual of Canine & Feline Wound Management and Reconstruction
Manual of Canine Practice: A Foundation Manual
Manual of Exotic Pet and Wildlife Nursing
Manual of Exotic Pets: A Foundation Manual
Manual of Feline Practice: A Foundation Manual
Manual of Ornamental Fish
Manual of Practical Animal Care
Manual of Practical Veterinary Nursing
Manual of Psittacine Birds
Manual of Rabbit Medicine
Manual of Rabbit Surgery, Dentistry and Imaging
Manual of Raptors, Pigeons and Passerine Birds
Manual of Reptiles
Manual of Rodents and Ferrets
Manual of Small Animal Practice Management and Development
Manual of Wildlife Casualties

For further information on these and all BSAVA publications, please visit
our website: **www.bsava.com**

Contents

Online extras

Downloadable forms

This Guide includes a series of downloadable forms to accompany the chapters, which are available from the BSAVA Library.

How to identify the forms in the text: in the selected chapters, the forms are identifiable by a 'download' symbol.

How to access the forms: the forms can be accessed using the QR code. You will need a QR code reader on your smart phone or tablet – a number of QR code readers apps are available. These forms can also be accessed by typing the web address **bsavalibrary.com/anaesthesiaforms** into a web browser.

Webinars and videos

A series of webinars and videos to accompany this Guide are being developed and will be available from the BSAVA Library. Email publications@bsava.com and we will contact you when videos become available. Use the QR code or type the web address **bsavalibrary.com/anaesthesiavideos** into a web browser to access these resources.

Foreword

As a practising anaesthetist involved in full time teaching of undergraduate, postgraduate and practising veterinary surgeons, I am always looking for ways to improve veterinary anaesthesia safety. Many factors influence the success of an anaesthetic procedure and eventually you begin to realise that paying attention to basic procedures and preparation has arguably the greatest impact on outcome. This has been exemplified by the aviation industry where cockpit checklists and procedures have dramatically improved the industry's safety record. The human anaesthetic field has also embraced this approach with similar positive outcomes.

With the diversity of veterinary anaesthetic practice around the world, introducing such rigid systems would not be feasible. However, with the help of this manual, basic safety checks could easily be introduced and adapted to the individual practice environment, potentially leading to significant reductions in adverse anaesthetic incidents. In addition, this handbook should be viewed as a 'second pair of eyes' when faced with stressful emergency situations when an anaesthetised patient deteriorates; consider it as having an experienced anaesthetist looking over your shoulder offering words of advice.

There is an enormous amount of experience within these pages and I am very happy to endorse this exciting new BSAVA resource.

Ian Self
BSc BVSc ARCS PGCertVetEd FHEA CertVA DipECVAA MRCVS
EBVS® European Veterinary Specialist in Veterinary Anaesthesia and Analgesia
RCVS Recognised Specialist in Veterinary Anaesthesia and Analgesia

Principal Clinical Anaesthetist
Affiliated Lecturer in Anaesthesia
Department of Veterinary Medicine
University of Cambridge
Madingley Road
Cambridge CB3 0ES

Preface

The primary aim for anyone working in veterinary medicine is to provide effective healthcare whilst minimizing harm to the patient. Progress has been made over recent years in terms of improved monitoring and pharmaceuticals, but the very real potential of anaesthesia causing harm remains. Anaesthesia, although considered routine by many, is a complex process involving a multitude of tasks that need to be performed in the correct way, in the correct order, at the correct time often in rapid succession. If any task in the process is missed or performed inappropriately the risk of harm to the patient increases. As such, anaesthesia lends itself to the application of cognitive aids.

Cognitive aids are visual prompts or decision guides, such as checklists or algorithms, which aim to reduce human error in critical processes by providing a supportive scaffolding that ensures tasks are performed and communicated appropriately. Unlike protocols or standard operating procedures, cognitive aids can be applied while a task is being performed. This reduces reliance on memory alone to perform tasks safely and effectively, and allows individuals to concentrate on other cognitive tasks, such as problem-solving and decision-making, while reducing the risk of cognitive overload, forgetfulness, distraction, fatigue or stress compromising the success of the task. They are particularly useful for critical steps that may not be readily recalled in high-pressure situations.

This guide can help reduce reliance on memory but it is neither a comprehensive step-by-step 'How to' guide for anaesthesia, nor an educational tool. It cannot prevent bad practice; ultimately, the onus to perform effective and safe anaesthesia remains with the individual and their team. Getting the most out of this guide will require familiarity with the content, engaging in practice sessions and applying checklists in clinics. However, it can hopefully help achieve the goal of providing our patients with the safest anaesthesia possible whatever the environment.

Matt McMillan
August 2020

Introduction and general information

Introduction

Cognitive aids, such as checklists, have a long history of improving safety in various industries, including aviation and nuclear power. More recently, their ability to improve safety in medicine has been established. The premise of a checklist is that it is very easy to forget a step in a process that is critical for this process to be performed effectively and safely in the heat of the moment (e.g. when under time pressure or in a life-or-death situation). Having a simple cognitive aid nearby can help reduce the chance of such safety-critical steps being missed.

Cognitive aids have been demonstrated to save lives and reduce incidence of complications such as postoperative infections. They have also been shown to improve team performance in crisis situations in operating theatres.

Cognitive aids are not there to tell you what to do or how to do it, rather they are there to reduce reliance on memory and to ensure that all the relevant tasks have been performed and considerations have been made.

Although cognitive aids can be used effectively by individuals, they are best used by a team. For them to be successful in this setting the entire team needs to be on board with their use. Training is essential to build effective teamwork.

Used properly, checklists can make your practice a safer place.

How to use this guide

These checklists are not intended to be an outline of standards of care. They should be used as cognitive aids not strict procedural policies.

Clinicians remain responsible for any decision regarding case management, which will depend on the animal's individual needs, the clinical data available, and the diagnostic and treatment options on offer.

Cognitive aids

Each cognitive aid is made up of a number of suggested checkpoints. Each numbered checkpoint is a task that should be carried out or considered before moving on to the next point. Tasks have been chosen as they are considered as critical safety steps or important considerations in the process that, if missed, risk injury to the animal. The checklists are designed to be used as **DO:CONFIRM, READ:DO** or '**mixed**' (see descriptions below), depending on the situation, how experienced the user is, and how well they know the checklist. It is important to recognize, even if you think you know these topics back to front, that anyone can miss out a step or make a misdiagnosis; therefore, a checklist should be utilized whenever problems are met that are not rapidly solved through memory and problem solving alone.

This guide is intended for use by trained staff who are familiar with it and who are practised in its use. It is worthwhile for all members of staff to become familiar with the format. Simulated training sessions using the checklists are recommended prior to use in clinical cases.

> ### DO:CONFIRM checklists
>
> These aids use natural pause points in a procedure; they are best employed for commonly performed routine tasks like setting up for an anaesthetic procedure (e.g. the anaesthetic safety checklists).
>
> The process is broken down into smaller distinct periods, which fit into natural breaks in a procedure's workflow (e.g. pre-induction, pre-procedure, and recovery).
>
> Each of these periods is broken down into smaller tasks.

DO:CONFIRM checklists *continued*

Typically, each task is performed (**DO**) from memory prior to running the checklist, in this way the checklist should not interfere with normal work patterns.

Prior to moving on to the next period of the process, each of the tasks should be read out loud and completion confirmed (**CONFIRM**), or the relevant information communicated. Any uncompleted tasks can then be performed prior to moving on.

READ:DO checklists

These aids are best used where there is uncertainty, for example, for new or not commonly performed tasks or where time is critical (e.g. crisis checklists).

Each point is read out (**READ**) before the task is then performed (**DO**).

MIXED DO:CONFIRM/READ:DO checklists

Often in an urgent situation people may have started a process (such as managing a hypotensive animal) prior to starting a checklist. This will be the case especially with experienced anaesthetists. In these cases, the checklist can act as **DO:CONFIRM** whilst you are checking off tasks that have been completed and **READ:DO** when uncompleted tasks are read out and then performed.

General cognitive aids

Section 2 contains general 'daily use' checklists and cognitive aids. These are designed to be used before, during and after each anaesthetic procedure, typically in the **DO:CONFIRM** format, concentrating on preparing the animal, equipment, drugs and veterinary team. They should be quick to run through for basic cases. However, for more complicated cases the checklists will be more involved in helping to ensure proper preparation and planning. They encourage communication and teamwork as well as helping ensure that no critical steps are missed in the process.

Each general checklist follows the same format:

- Guideline name
- When the checklist should be performed
- Numbered considerations to be made and/or tasks to be performed before moving on in the process.

Crisis cognitive aids

In **Section 3**, there are a set of cognitive aids for crisis situations. If a crisis has been identified it is always wise to run through a quick assessment prior to starting interventions, which ensures aspects of the situation are not overlooked (see **Rapid situational assessment**). This assessment should allow for a specific crisis to be identified.

On completion, the team can move on to the appropriate crisis checklists. A diagnostic table is available to help with diagnosis. Crisis checklists are best used in a **READ:DO** or **mixed** format. Again, the checklists are there to support communication and decision making, not to define them.

Each crisis checklist follows the same format:

- Guideline name
- A brief description of the clinical situation for which the guideline is written
- The objective of the checklist
- Numbered considerations to be made and/or tasks to be performed
- Bullet points to help identify sub-category tasks and considerations.

How to run the checklists

Each checklist should be used in the same simple way:

- Work through the numbered points in order
- Ideally someone (not the person performing the tasks) should read the point aloud
- This person should ensure that each task is performed, each point is considered, and that steps are not missed out.

In the case of a crisis checklist, if a problem worsens or fails to respond, the **Rapid situational assessment** checklist should be performed again, whilst taking into consideration the general and crisis-specific diagnostic tables.

Section 2:

General cognitive aids

Pre-anaesthetic assessment

1. Clinical history

- What are the animal's current problems?
- Is the animal eating, drinking, urinating and defecating normally?
- When did the animal last eat and drink?
- Has the animal lost any weight?
- Does the animal have a history of vomiting or regurgitation?
- Has the animal been coughing, sneezing or had any problems breathing (including audible respiratory noise)?
- Has the animal been exercising well/normally?
- Is the animal taking any current medications?
- Has the animal had previous anaesthetics?
- If so, were any problems reported or seen by owner on recovery?

2. Clinical examination
Pay special attention to:

- Major body systems:
  - Cardiovascular
  - Respiratory (including airway)
  - Neurological
  - Abdominal organs
- Patient size, body condition and conformation (e.g. brachycephalic airway issues)
- Temperament and behaviour (e.g. anxiety, aggression)
- Current pain state
- Body temperature.

3. Signalment
Will the animal's signalment pose any problems? Consider:

- Age
- Species
- Breed
- Sex.

4. Procedural considerations

What problems might the procedure pose? Consider:

- Pain
- Haemorrhage
- Interference with vital structures (heart, lungs, major abdominal viscera, nerves)
- Logistics (e.g. access to animal).

5. Anaesthetic considerations

Will anything from the above likely increase the chance of adverse events occurring? Consider:

- Hypotension
- Hypoventilation
- Hypoxaemia
- Hypo- or hyperthermia
- Arousal (e.g. moving animal between multiple locations, extremely painful points of a procedure, hyperthermia/pyrexia increasing anaesthetic requirements)
- Bradycardia
- Tachycardia
- Other arrhythmia.

6. Other considerations

Including (but not limited to):

- Is the animal going to have problems metabolizing drugs (very young, very old, very sick or those with hepatic impairment)?
- Will any of the medications the animal is on interact with any drugs that could potentially be administered during the anaesthetic period?
- Is fasting likely to adversely affect the patient (e.g. very young, diabetic)?

Section 1

Section 2

Section 3

Anaesthetic planning questions

1. **Has anything significant been identified in the history and/or clinical examination?**

2. **Do any abnormalities warrant further investigation?**

3. **Can any abnormalities be stabilized prior to anaesthesia?**

4. **What complications are anticipated during anaesthesia?**

5. **How can these complications be managed?**

6. **What type of premedication would the patient benefit from?**

7. **How will any pain associated with the procedure be managed?**

8. **How will anaesthesia be induced and maintained?**

9. **How readily can the animal be intubated?**

10. **How will the patient be monitored?**

11. **How will the patient's body temperature be maintained?**

12. **How will the patient be positioned?**

13. **How will the patient be managed in the post-anaesthetic period?**

14. **Are the required facilities, personnel and drugs available?**

Essential drugs

Anaesthetics, sedatives and analgesics

1. Sedatives:
- Acepromazine
- Dexmedetomidine or medetomidine
- Diazepam or midazolam.

2. Opioids:
- Methadone
- Buprenorphine
- Butorphanol (for non-painful procedures)
- *Useful but not essential: fentanyl.*

3. Induction and maintenance agents:
- Alfaxalone or propofol
- Isoflurane or sevoflurane.

4. Additional analgesics:
- Non-steroidal anti-inflammatory drugs (carprofen, meloxicam or robenacoxib)
- Ketamine
- Lidocaine
- *Useful but not essential: bupivacaine or ropivacaine.*

Emergency and therapeutic drugs

5. Cardiovascular and respiratory drugs:
- Atropine
- Adrenaline
- Ephedrine
- Lidocaine without adrenaline
- Salbutamol (inhaler)
- *Useful but not essential: dobutamine, dopamine, glycopyrrolate, noradrenaline, terbutaline.*

Essential drugs *continued*

6. Other:

- Atipamezole
- Calcium borogluconate
- Chlorphenamine
- Dexamethasone
- Glucose 50%
- Maropitant
- Metoclopramide
- *Desired: naloxone (in case of full agonist opioid overdose)*
- *Useful but not essential: omeprazole, sodium bicarbonate.*

Anaesthetic machine checklist

1. **Primary oxygen source checked**

2. **Back-up oxygen available**

3. **Oxygen alarm working (if present)**

4. **Flowmeters working**

5. **Vaporizer attached, locked and full**

6. **Anaesthetic machine passed leak test**

7. **Scavenging checked**

8. **Available monitoring equipment functioning**

9. **Airway equipment checked**

10. **Emergency equipment and drugs checked**

11. **Breathing systems available and checked**

Breathing system checklist

1. Visually inspect breathing system

- Tubes and reservoir bag intact.
- No foreign bodies in the tubes.
- Adjustable pressure-limiting (APL) valve opens and closes.
- For rebreathing systems: soda lime is not exhausted.

2. Attach breathing system to anaesthetic machine and scavenging system

3. Perform a leak test

Occlusion test for non-rebreathing systems:

- Occlude the breathing system at the patient connector
- Close the APL valve
- Fill the system with O_2 until the bag is 'tight'
- Turn off the O_2
- Ensure system maintains pressure and volume
- Safety APL valves should open at high pressures when the bag is squeezed
- For co-axial systems (e.g. Bain) perform an occlusion test on the inner tube
- Open the APL valve
- Ensure gas is able to freely leave the APL valve.

Two-bag test for circle breathing systems:

- Attach a spare reservoir bag to the patient connector
- Close the APL valve and set a fresh gas flow of 5 l/min
- Check the one-way valves by squeezing each bag in turn
- Check the APL valve by squeezing both bags
- Turn off fresh gas and fill the system using O_2 flush until the bags are full (if a manometer is used, set a system pressure of 30 cmH_2O)
- Ensure system maintains pressure and volume
- Open the APL valve
- Ensure gas is able to freely leave the APL valve.

4. Ensure the APL valve is fully open

Essential equipment checklist

Are the following readily available?

1. Ability to gain intravenous access

2. Ability to administer oxygen

3. Induction and maintenance

4. Ability to gain an airway
- Endotracheal tubes (cuffs checked).
- Airway aids (e.g. guidewire, laryngoscope, suction).

5. Ability to provide a positive-pressure breath
- Self-inflating bag (e.g. Ambu-bag).
- Bain, T-piece or circle breathing system with reservoir bag.

6. Ability to provide fluid therapy
- Isotonic crystalloid solution.
- Fluid giving set.

7. Ability to provide physiological monitoring
- Trained personnel.
- Oesophageal stethoscope.
- Pulse oximetry.
- Capnography.
- Thermometer.
- Doppler or oscillometric blood pressure.
- Electrocardiogram.

8. Warming devices to help patient maintain body temperature

9. Ability to rapidly administer emergency drugs

10. Ability to administer basic life support

Difficult airway equipment checklist

10

1. **Range of endotracheal tubes ready**

2. **Laryngoscope with working light source and appropriate blade sizes ready**

3. **Guidewires, stylet, male urinary catheter ready**

4. **'Cuff syringe' ready**

5. **Tube tie ready**

6. **Suction ready**

7. **Capnograph (if available) turned on**

8. **Pulse oximeter turned on and, if possible, attached to patient**

9. **Breathing system for pre-oxygenation ready**

10. **Additional induction agent ready**

11. **Surgical airway kit ready**

12. **Appropriate personnel available**

13. **Plan communicated**

Crash box

1. Syringes and needles
- Range of syringes with needles attached.

2. Self-inflating bag (Ambu-bag)

3. Adrenaline
- Can be drawn up pre-diluted 1:10 with saline (requires altered drug chart).

4. Atropine

5. Drug chart and cardiopulmonary resuscitation (CPR) algorithm

6. Airway equipment
- Full range of endotracheal tubes.
- Laryngoscope.
- Tube tie.

Safety checklist: pre-induction

1. **Confirm patient's name**

2. **Confirm procedure to be performed**

3. **Confirm client consent obtained**

4. **Intravenous access patent?**

5. **Airway equipment ready**

6. **Anaesthetic machine ready**

7. **Breathing system ready**

8. **Are antibiotics required?**

9. **Likely complications communicated**

10. **Plan confirmed**

Post-induction checklist

1. Oxygen on
Set to an adequate flow for the size of the animal and the type of breathing system.

2. Airway
Confirm placement of the endotracheal tube:

- Visual confirmation
- Capnograph trace
- Reservoir bag moving when patient breathes
- Chest moves during administration of positive-pressure breaths.

3. Breathing
- Confirm appropriate chest wall and abdominal movements.
- Confirm the reservoir bag is moving and the breathing system is intact.

4. Circulation
- Manually palpate peripheral pulse.

5. Depth
- Confirm depth of anaesthesia.

6. Check essential electronic monitoring
- Pulse oximetry – confirm oxygen saturation (SpO_2) over 95%.
- Capnography – confirm trace.

7. Inflate endotracheal tube cuff
- For polyvinyl chloride (PVC) tubes ideally use a cuff manometer device.
- Alternatively, use a 'loss of leak' technique:
  - Listen for a leak at the animal's mouth
  - Administer a slow, low pressure positive-pressure manual breath
  - Inflate the cuff until no leak is audible.

8. Start general anaesthetic agent

Safety checklist: before starting procedure

1. **Confirm animal's name**

2. **Confirm procedure, plan and personnel**

3. **Antibiotics administered if necessary**

4. **Swab count confirmed**

5. **All equipment ready**

6. **Safety concerns communicated**

7. **Anaesthetic depth confirmed**

8. **Ask: can we start?**

Safety checklist: before recovery

1. **Have all the necessary procedures been performed?**

2. **Are all swabs accounted for?**

3. **Are all sharps and instruments accounted for?**

4. **Have all throat packs/purse-string sutures been removed?**

5. **Are all samples labelled and safe?**

6. **Safety concerns communicated**
   Including (but not limited to):
   - Airway
   - Breathing
   - Circulation and fluid balance
   - Pain
   - Temperature.

7. **Recovery plan confirmed**
   Including (but not limited to):
   - Analgesia plan
   - Fluid therapy
   - Nutrition
   - Wound care (e.g. drains, surgical site)
   - Sedation
   - Management of clinical signs (e.g. anti-nausea medication).

Recovery and patient handover checklist

1. **Animal name and signalment**

2. **Details of procedure**

3. **Outline of problems**
   - Pre-existing diagnoses.
   - With procedure.
   - With anaesthetic.

4. **Details of relevant management**
   - How problems are dealt with.

5. **Outline of current status**
   - Overall.
   - Last body temperature measurement.

6. **Outline of plan**
   - Analgesia.
   - Other medications.
   - Likely complications.
   - Monitoring and assessments.
   - When to be concerned.
   - Interventions.

7. **Confirm who to call in an emergency**

8. **Any questions?**

Section 3:

Crisis checklists and cognitive aids

Section 1

Section 2

Section 3

Rapid situational assessment

1. Communicate

- Alert team to the concern.

2. Ensure adequate oxygen supply

- Flowmeter working.
- Flow set to adequate level.
- Oxygen pressure 4 kPa and cylinder pressure adequate (not in the red).

3. Check pulses and breathing

- Start cardiopulmonary resuscitation (CPR) if necessary.

4. Ventilate

Administer one manual breath to confirm:

- No airway resistance
- Airway patent
- Breathing system patent – no leak
- Capnograph trace present
- Chest wall moves
- Lung compliance good (does the pressure in the bag feel normal given the amount you have squeezed the bag?)
- Lung sounds present.

5. Check anaesthetic depth

6. Check all monitoring resources and equipment

7. Check on procedure status

- Blood loss.
- Pressure on organs, diaphragm or blood vessels.

8. Check intravenous access and all infusion lines

9. Check and adjust all drugs

- Alter vaporizer setting as appropriate.
- Administer bolus of injectable agent if the animal is moving or likely to move.

10. Review and evaluate all information

Cross-reference findings:

- Does everything fit?
- Is everything in agreement?
- Does anything stand out?

11. Identify crisis type and start considering diagnoses

12. Go to relevant checklist

Diagnostic considerations

Problem	Signs	Potential causes
Increased abdominal pressure	Mixed cardiovascular and respiratory effects: tachycardia and hypotension; hypoventilation and hypoxaemia	Gastric or intestinal dilatation, torsion of viscus, pregnancy, abdominal organ enlargement, bladder distension, surgical pressure
Airway failure	Exaggerated attempts to breathe, little or no movement of reservoir bag, true apnoea	Kinked or dislodged endotracheal (ET) tube, aspiration, blockage of ET tube
Anaphylaxis	Hypotension, tachycardia, obstructed capnograph trace (indicates bronchospasm), urticaria	Any drugs (antibiotics), transfused blood products, human albumin
Calcium abnormalities	Hypercalcaemia: arrhythmia	Renal, hyperparathyroidism, toxicity, paraneoplastic
	Hypocalcaemia: tachycardia, arrhythmia	Acidosis, toxicity, inflammatory disease, pregnancy
Cardiac	Arrhythmia, hypotension, poor pulse quality	Primary: occult cardiac disease, myocardial or valvular dysfunction
		Secondary: abdominal disease (splenic disease, inflammation) leading to arrhythmia
		Electrolyte abnormalities
Embolus	Hypotension, sudden hypocapnia, arrhythmia	Air, fat, thrombus or bone cement lodges in pulmonary vasculature Seen: • When surgical site above level of right atrium (e.g. hemilaminectomy, limb surgery, amputation) • During orthopaedic surgery (e.g. fracture repair, total hip replacement) • If excess air in fluid lines

Problem	Signs	Potential causes
Endocrine	Hypertension, tachyarrhythmia	Hyperthyroidism
	Hypotension, bradycardia	Hypothyroidism or hypoadrenocorticism
	Hypotension with either tachycardia or bradycardia	Diabetes mellitus
Equipment malfunction	Multiple depending on equipment	Oxygen delivery failure, breathing system failure; adjustable pressure-limiting (APL) valve closed, tubing kinked, fluid pump failure
Fluid balance	Tachycardia, hypotension, poor pulse quality, pale mucous membranes, slow capillary refill time	Hypovolaemia
	Increased respiratory effort, altered lung sounds	Fluid overload
Hypoglycaemia	Bradycardia, hypotension, hypothermia, inappropriately deep plane of anaesthesia, delayed recovery	Liver dysfunction, insulin, paraneoplastic, neonate, sepsis
Intravenous access	Failure to respond as expected to intravenous drug administration	Cannula no longer patent (clot, kink), cannula dislodged
Inflammatory	Poorly responsive hypotension	Sepsis, systemic inflammatory response syndrome (SIRS)
Potassium abnormalities	Hyperkalaemia: bradycardia, arrhythmia	Acute kidney injury, urethral obstruction, urinary tract rupture, hypoadrenocorticism, cell lysis, over-administration of potassium supplementation
	Hypokalaemia: muscle weakness, tachycardia, arrhythmia	Inappetence, fluid therapy, renal losses, gastrointestinal losses
Respiratory disease	Tachypnoea, hypoxaemia, dyspnoea	Underlying respiratory disease: • Oedema • Pneumonia • Lower airway disease • Neoplasia • Contusion • Atelectasis

»

Section 1

Section 2

Section 3

Diagnostic considerations *continued*

Problem	Signs	Potential causes
Temperature regulation	Hypothermia: bradycardia, hypotension, low respiratory rate and hypocapnia, increased depth of anaesthesia	High surface area:volume ratio, failure of heating device, large exposed surgical field
	Hyperthermia: tachycardia, hypertension, tachypnoea, decreased depth of anaesthesia	Pre-anaesthetic hyperthermia: large hairy dogs on hot days, seizures, pyrexia, activity, stress, airway or respiratory problems Malignant hyperthermia
Transfusion reaction	Haemoglobinaemia, icterus, hypotension, tachycardia, bronchospasm, urticaria	Transfusion reaction to blood products, albumin or colloids
Traumatic injuries	Any respiratory or cardiovascular abnormalities	Pulmonary or cardiac contusions, pneumothorax, ruptured bladder, occult haemorrhage
Weight	Mixed: often hypotension and ventilation/oxygenation issues	Diaphragmatic splinting, caval compression, reduced functional residual capacity

Cardiopulmonary arrest and basic life support

Description:	Pulseless or gasping patient
Objective:	Return of spontaneous circulation, identify and correct cause

1. Call for help

2. Intubate if not already

3. Start cardiopulmonary resuscitation (CPR) cycle (2 min)

- Turn off anaesthetic agent and stop all drugs.
- Start compressions:
    - 100–120 per min, half chest width, full chest recoil, lateral recumbency
    - For cats and small dogs <10 kg, compress over heart (barrel-chested dogs <10 kg may benefit from compressions over the widest part of the thorax)
    - For medium to large dogs >10 kg, compress over widest part of thorax.
- Start ventilation:
    - 10 breaths/min, 10 ml/kg, 1 second inspiratory time.
- Initiate monitoring:
    - Electrocardiogram (ECG), end-tidal carbon dioxide (ET'CO$_2$) (aim for >15 mmHg).
- Antagonize drugs.
- Consider adrenaline and atropine:
    - Only if this does not distract from chest compressions.
- Evaluate potential underlying problems and act accordingly.

Nearest location for **Adrenaline**

Nearest location for **Atropine**

Cardiopulmonary and basic life support
continued

4. End of CPR cycle (take 5 seconds maximum)

- Change person doing compressions.
- Check ECG/evaluate animal.
- Restart CPR cycle at point (3).

5. Stop after:

- Consciousness or cranial nerve reflexes return
  - Good sign of effective oxygen delivery
- Spontaneous circulation returns
- Spontaneous breathing returns
- 15–30 minutes of no success.

Cardiopulmonary resuscitation (CPR) drugs chart

Weight	Drug (Dose)		
	Adrenaline – low 1:1000 (0.01 mg/kg)	Adrenaline – high 1:1000 (0.1 mg/kg)	Atropine 0.6 mg/ml (0.04 mg/kg)
1 kg	0.01 ml	0.1 ml	0.07 ml
2 kg	0.02 ml	0.2 ml	0.14 ml
3 kg	0.03 ml	0.3 ml	0.2 ml
4 kg	0.04 ml	0.4 ml	0.27 ml
5 kg	0.05 ml	0.5 ml	0.33 ml
10 kg	0.1 ml	1.0 ml	0.7 ml
15 kg	0.15 ml	1.5 ml	1.0 ml
20 kg	0.2 ml	2.0 ml	1.3 ml
25 kg	0.25 ml	2.5 ml	1.7 ml
30 kg	0.3 ml	3.0 ml	2.0 ml
35 kg	0.35 ml	3.5 ml	2.3 ml
40 kg	0.4 ml	4.0 ml	2.7 ml
45 kg	0.45 ml	4.5 ml	3.0 ml
50 kg	0.5 ml	5.0 ml	3.3 ml

Note: Dilute adrenaline 1:10 with saline

Difficult airway

Description: Difficulties placing endotracheal tube or supraglottic airway. Common in brachycephalic animals or animals with orofacial problems, following laryngospasm, and in difficult to intubate species such as rabbits

Objective: Maintain haemoglobin oxygen saturation (SpO_2) whilst gaining an airway

1. **Call for help**

2. **Administer high-flow oxygen via facemask**
   - Hand ventilate if the animal is not breathing.

3. **Monitor saturation**
   - Hand ventilate via facemask if SpO_2 level drops below 93–95%.

4. **Optimize intubation conditions**
   - Optimize body, head and neck position.
   - Laryngoscope or instrument to depress tongue and light source.
   - Suction as necessary.
   - Array of endotracheal tubes.
   - Stylet or guidewire or male dog urinary catheter.
   - Topical local anaesthetic.
   - Ensure adequate depth of anaesthesia.
   - Administer analgesia if there are problems opening the mouth.

5. **Reattempt intubation**
   - If the larynx can be visualized, consider placing a guidewire or stylet.
   - A male dog urinary catheter can be connected to a syringe barrel attached to an endotracheal tube connector and used to insufflate oxygen.
   - Use this to guide endotracheal tube.

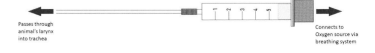

Passes through animal's larynx into trachea

Connects to Oxygen source via breathing system

6. Consider aborting procedure if safe to do so or obtain a surgical airway

- Provide oxygen via mask ventilation or via urinary catheter as described above.
- Antagonize drugs if aborting and recovering from anaesthesia.

Post-induction apnoea

Description:	Cessation in spontaneous respiration following intravenous induction. Common especially if induction agent is administered too rapidly
Objective:	Adequately ventilate the lungs, restore spontaneous ventilation

1. Confirm pulses

■ Start cardiopulmonary resuscitation (CPR) if necessary.

2. Hand ventilate

■ Administer two positive-pressure breaths.

■ Airway patent? End-tidal carbon dioxide (ET'CO$_2$) trace visualized? Chest moves with intermittent positive-pressure ventilation? Endotracheal tube cuff leaking?

3. Assess anaesthetic depth

■ If depth appropriate or 'too deep', may be able to wait.

■ If depth 'too light', start isoflurane and give two more breaths then reassess.

4. Check oxygen saturation (SpO$_2$)

■ Monitor and administer two positive-pressure breaths if below 93–95%.

5. Monitor ET'CO$_2$

■ If SpO$_2$ remains above 93–95% administer two positive-pressure breaths per minute allowing ET'CO$_2$ to increase up to 50–55 mmHg to stimulate spontaneous respiration.

6. If not successful start mechanical ventilation

Hypoxaemia, desaturation and cyanosis

| Description: | Drop in oxygen saturation (SpO_2) <93% or partial pressure of oxygen (P_aO_2) <60 mmHg or a P_aO_2: fraction of inspired oxygen (FiO_2) of <200 |
| Objective: | Restore adequate oxygenation |

Warning: Always assume pulse oximeters are accurate if hypoxaemia is likely

Pay special attention if there is a history, clinical findings or differential diagnosis of:

- Pulmonary disease
- Lower airway disease
- Upper airway disease or dysfunction
- Coughing
- Traumatic injury
- Abdominal enlargement
- Breathing difficulties
- Regurgitation or vomiting
- Aspiration.

1. Ensure FiO_2 100%

- Check oxygen source.
- Oxygen concentrator working (oxygen meter confirming FiO_2).
- Flowmeters working.

2. Hand ventilate

- Is the airway patent?
- Check for obstructions – listen for gurgling from the airway (airway secretions, haemorrhage, kinks in tubing)
- Is the breathing system patent and sealed – listen for a hissing sound or is there loss of volume/pressure in system?
- Is the chest moving?
- Is resistance/compliance normal?

≫

Hypoxaemia, desaturation and cyanosis *continued*

2. Hand ventilate *continued*

- Is there a capnograph trace?
- Consider accidental endobronchial intubation? How long was the endotracheal tube?

3. Auscultate chest

- Are there lung sounds present on both sides?
- Any unusual lung sounds?

4. Check signal quality

- Move probe.
- Ensure good pulse signal.

5. Ensure adequate perfusion

- Assess blood pressure, pulse quality and heart rate.
- See **Hypotension** checklist.

6. Consider:

- Suctioning the airway
- Re-intubating
- Changing breathing system
- Reducing depth of anaesthesia
- Administering salbutamol via an inhaler
- Diagnostic imaging – thoracic radiography and ultrasonography
- Terminating procedure
- Recruitment manoeuvre and instigating positive-end expiratory pressure
- Arterial blood gas analysis.

Nearest location for **Suction**

Causes of hypoxaemia and desaturation

Low fraction of inspired oxygen (FiO_2)

- Oxygen source failed

Hypoventilation

- Post-induction apnoea
- Inappropriate depth of anaesthesia
- Pharmacological (opioids, ketamine, muscle relaxants)
- Airway obstruction
- Low functional residual capacity (obesity, pregnancy, abdominal distension, diaphragmatic splinting, pleural space)
- Panting
- Cervical spinal disease
- Neuromuscular disease

Diffusion barrier impairment

- Fibrotic lung disease (old terriers especially West Highland White Terriers and cats with chronic feline asthma syndrome)

Ventilation/perfusion mismatch (V:Q mismatch)

- Oedema: protein rich (acute lung injury, acute respiratory distress syndrome, transfusion-related acute lung injury, inflammatory disease, neurogenic); protein free (fluid overload, left-sided heart failure)
- Haemorrhage: pulmonary contusions, coagulopathy
- Atelectasis: prolonged recumbency, diaphragmatic splinting, pleural space disease, obesity, neuromuscular blocking agent, prolonged anaesthesia with 100% O_2
- Hypotension
- Airway disease: asthma, bronchial disease
- Other: pus (bronchopneumonia, aspirated fluid)

Interpulmonary shunt

- Congenital cardiac disease: patent ductus arteriosis, patent foramen ovale, septal defects
- Neoplasia
- Severe pulmonary diseases

Hypotension

Description:	Drop in blood pressure (suggested threshold mean arterial pressure 60 mmHg, systolic arterial pressure 80 mmHg). Inability to obtain blood pressure measurements, weak/absent peripheral pulses
Objective:	Restore haemodynamic stability

If there is haemorrhage, anaphylaxis, tachycardia or bradycardia, see relevant checklists.

1. Check pulses

- Start cardiopulmonary resuscitation if required.

2. Confirm hypotension

- Re-measure blood pressure.

3. Reduce vaporizer setting

- Assess anaesthetic depth.
- Reduce vaporizer setting and consider altering anaesthetic protocol (e.g. increase analgesia, add in intravenous agents or switch to total intravenous anaesthesia).

4. Assess heart rate

- If low, consider treating for primary bradycardia:
  - Atropine: 0.02–0.04 mg/kg or
  - Glycopyrrolate: 0.1 mg/kg (unlicensed).
- If high, consider hypovolaemia, arrhythmia, poor contractility or vasodilatory states.

Nearest location for **Atropine**

5. Consider administering fluid bolus

- Exercise caution in animals with heart disease, respiratory disease and where hypovolaemia is unlikely.
- Respiratory pulse profile variation (especially following positive-pressure ventilation) may indicate likely fluid responsiveness (see below).
- Administer 10–30 ml/kg isotonic crystalloid (lactated Ringer's solution or 0.9% NaCl) or 2–5 ml/kg colloid in dogs and assess response. Use 5–10 ml/kg isotonic crystalloid or 1–2 ml/kg colloid in cats and assess response.

Respiratory pulse profile variation
Following a positive-pressure breath, if a significant (>15%) drop in pulse profile (e.g. on a pulse oximeter plethysmograph) occurs (see arrow in diagram) the hypotension will likely respond to fluid boluses

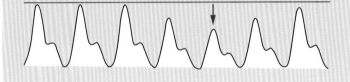

6. Consider pharmacological support

- Ephedrine 50–100 μg/kg q20min up to 3 times
- Noradrenaline* 0.1–1 μg/kg/min
- Dopamine* 5–20 μg/kg/min
- Dobutamine* 1–10 μg/kg/min
- Adrenaline* 0.1–2 μg/kg/min
- Phenylephrine* 2–10 μg/kg q5–15min or 0.1–1 μg/kg/min.

Direct arterial blood pressure monitoring advisable when using these drugs.

Nearest location for **Ephedrine**

Hypotension *continued*

Causes of hypotension
Haemorrhage
• Blood in site • Blood in suction • Blood on swabs • Blood on table/floor/hidden by drapes • Occult bleeding – history of trauma?
Hypovolaemia of other cause
• Large swing in pulse profile following a positive-pressure breath • History of pre-anaesthetic volume deficit
Vasodilation
• Excessive anaesthetic administration • Acepromazine administered in premedication • Systemic inflammatory response syndrome/sepsis • Vagal stimulation • Anaphylaxis – bronchoconstriction/urticaria • Release of vasoactive substance
Obstruction
• Vascular compression (e.g. surgeon) • Mass effect (e.g. obesity, pregnancy, organomegaly)
Poor cardiac contractility
• Myocardial diseases (e.g. cardiomyopathy) • Drug-related • Disease-related (e.g. hypothyroidism, critical illness) • Age-related (paediatric or geriatric)
Arrhythmia
• Bradycardia – 'too slow to flow' (e.g. sinus bradycardia, atrioventricular block) • Tachycardia – 'too fast to fill' (e.g. ventricular tachycardia, atrial fibrillation, supraventricular tachycardia)
Other
• Rapid removal of a chronic abdominal effusion • Ligation of a major blood vessel (e.g. patent ductus arteriosis, portosytemic shunt, renal vein) • Sudden change in body position (e.g. sternal to dorsal)

Bronchoconstriction

Description: Sudden increase in expiratory effort, shark fin capnograph trace, audible wheezing on expiration when auscultated, may be accompanied by hypoxaemia. Often following intubation or bronchoalveolar lavage

Objective: Cause bronchodilation which is maintained into recovery

1. Ensure fraction of inspired oxygen (FiO₂) 100%

2. Ensure upper airway patent

- Place endotracheal (ET) tube if not intubated (use local anaesthetic on larynx to avoid laryngospasm).
- Check ET tube for kinks.
- Check breathing system for kinks or obstructions.
- If in doubt, change the ET tube (especially in cats or brachycephalic animals).

3. Check for anaphylaxis

- Swollen face.
- Urticaria.
- Hypotension.
- Tachycardia.

4. Consider the following bronchodilators:

- Isoflurane or sevoflurane
- Ketamine 0.5–1 mg/kg i.v.
- Lidocaine 2 mg/kg given over 2–3 minutes (dogs only)
- Terbutaline 0.01 mg/kg i.m. or i.v.
- Salbutamol inhaler 100 µg per 'puff':
  - 1 puff for small-sized animals
  - 2 for medium-sized animals
  - 3 for large-sized animals
- Adrenaline 1–10 µg/kg (0.01 mg/kg diluted given to effect i.v.).

5. Consider terminating the procedure

6. Monitor on recovery for reoccurrence of bronchoconstriction

Haemorrhage

Description: Massive uncontrolled blood loss
Objective: Maintain perfusion to major organs whilst minimizing haemorrhage and coagulopathy until haemorrhage is controlled. Restore haemodynamic stability

1. Control haemorrhage

- Tourniquet, pressure, clamp, haemostatic dressings.

2. Fluid boluses

- Bolus isotonic crystalloid (Hartmann's or 0.9% NaCl, preferably warmed) 10–30 ml/kg in dogs and 5–15 ml/kg in cats.
- Repeat as necessary.
- Intend to administer isotonic crystalloid at 1:1 to 2:1 of blood volume lost.
- 90 ml/kg = blood volume in a dog; 60 ml/kg = blood volume in a cat.

3. Reduce vaporizer setting

- Reduce and consider altering the anaesthetic protocol (e.g. increase analgesia, initiate supplemental intravenous drugs).

4. Estimate loss

- Weigh swabs, volume in suction (calculate dilution), volume on table/floor.

5. Blood products

- Assessment for the use of blood products should be performed on a case-by-case cost:benefit basis.
- Suggested potential transfusion triggers:
  - If following appropriate fluid resuscitation packed cell volume is likely to be <20% or haemoglobin 7 g/dl in dogs; <15% or 5 g/dl in cats; or
  - >30–50% blood loss.
- Fresh whole blood ideal (contains platelets).
- Otherwise fresh frozen plasma and packed red blood cells 1:1.

Nearest location for **Blood products**

6. Hypotensive resuscitation

■ Consider if unable to control haemorrhage.

■ Maintain blood pressure between 50–60 mmHg (mean) or 70–90 mmHg (systolic) or just palpable peripheral pulses (reduces ongoing blood loss and allows easier resolution of bleeding).

7. Maintain normothermia

■ Hypothermia = coagulopathy.

■ Warm patient, environment, lavage and fluids.

8. Consider coagulopathy

■ Continued oozing at surgical sites.

■ Fresh frozen plasma (10–15 ml/kg) or consider cryoprecipitate for von Willebrand's Factor and Factor VIII.

■ Tranexamic acid 10 mg/kg (unlicensed).

Hypertension

Description: Sudden increase in blood pressure, systolic arterial pressure >160 mmHg
Objective: Restore normotension

1. Check heart rate

- Hypertension + tachycardia could indicate pain or inadequate depth of anaesthesia or sympathetic storm.
- Hypertension + bradycardia could indicate raised intracranial pressure or response to alpha-2 agonists.

2. Stop and/or antagonize vasoconstrictors

- Atipamezole for dogs at:
  - 5 times medetomidine dose (same volume)
  - 10 times dexmedetomidine dose (same volume).
- Atipamezole for cats at:
  - 2.5 times medetomidine dose (half volume)
  - 5 times dexmedetomidine dose (half volume).
- Stop adrenergic agents (e.g. noradrenaline, adrenaline, phenylephrine, dopamine, dobutamine).
  - This may lighten the plane of anaesthetic so check anaesthetic depth regularly.

Nearest location for **Atipamezole**

3. Ensure appropriate anaesthetic depth

- Check and correct if required.

4. Ensure analgesia optimized

- Opioids:
  - Fentanyl 1–5 µg/kg
  - Methadone 0.1 mg/kg (may need intermittent positive-pressure ventilation).

Section 1

Section 2

Section 3

- Lidocaine 1–2 mg/kg slow i.v.
- Consider patient body position – especially old patients with degenerative joint disease (elbow/hip position).

5. **Consider administering vasodilators:**

- Consider deliberately deepening anaesthesia
- Consider acepromazine 5–10 µg/kg
- Consider magnesium 40–50 mg/kg over 15 minutes then 15 mg/kg/h
- Consider phentolamine 0.02–0.1 µg/kg then 1–2 µg/kg/min
- Consider nitroprusside 0.5–15 µg/kg/min.

Bradycardia

Description:	Sudden decrease in heart rate or heart rate <60 bpm in dogs and <100 bpm in cats
Objective:	Ensure adequate perfusion. Increase heart rate if required

1. **Confirm pulses**

2. **Pause surgical manipulations**

3. **Check blood pressure:**
   - Is the heart rate affecting perfusion pressure (mean arterial pressure <60 mmHg, systolic arterial pressure <80 mmHg)? **OR**
   - Is heart rate an effect of blood pressure (baroreceptor reflex)?
     - May be a side effect of alpha-2 agonists (heart rate may be acceptable if blood pressure good)
     - If high, see **Hypertension** checklist.

4. **Check electrocardiogram**
   - Can you identify the rhythm?

5. **Check anaesthetic depth**
   - Reduce vaporizer setting if necessary.
   - Especially relevant if the patient is hypothermic as hypothermia increases depth of anaesthesia.

6. **Consider electrolyte abnormalities**
   - Is an electrolyte disturbance likely (K^+ or Ca^{2+})?
   - If yes, check and correct as required.

7. **Consider pharmacological intervention**
   - Antagonize alpha-2 agonists:
     - Atipamezole for dogs at:
       - 5 times medetomidine dose (same volume)
       - 10 times dexmedetomidine dose (same volume).
     - Atipamezole for cats at:
       - 2.5 times medetomidine dose (half volume)
       - 5 times dexmedetomidine dose (half volume).

Nearest location for **Atipamezole**

- Anticholinergics:
  - Atropine 20–50 µg/kg
  - Glycopyrrolate 5–10 µg/kg
  - May cause reflex bradycardia before heart rate increases.

Nearest location for **Atropine**

- Adrenergic agents:
  - Useful in hypothermic patients
  - Ephedrine 50–100 µg/kg
  - Adrenaline 1–10 µg/kg diluted given slowly to effect.

8. Warm hypothermic patients
- Warm patient, environment, lavage and fluids.

Causes of bradycardia
Vagally mediated
• Pharmacological (opioids and alpha-2 agonists) • Reflex or surgical manipulation or sudden change in body position (e.g. oculovagal, trigeminal-vagal, vagovagal, vasovagal, baroreceptor, cranial abdomen, cardiovagal, Bezold-Jarisch reflex)
Hypothermia
• Any cause (especially with hypovolaemia in cats)
Primary arrhythmia
• Atrioventricular block (3rd degree) or sick sinus syndrome
Hyperkalaemia
• Acute kidney injury • Urinary bladder rupture or urethral blockage • Hypoadrenocorticism (Addison's disease) • Cellular (e.g. reperfusion injury, massive trauma, haemolysis) • Inadvertent rapid administration of fluids supplemented with potassium chloride
Hypercalcaemia
• Pathophysiological (e.g. paraneoplastic, renal, hyperparathyroidism) • Toxicity
Raised intracranial pressure
• Cushing's reflex (hypertension, bradycardia, respiratory abnormalities)
Local anaesthetic toxicity
• Potential of overdose if >4 mg/kg lidocaine, 2 mg/kg bupivacaine or i.v. administration

Tachycardia

Description:	Sudden elevation in heart rate or heart rate >180 bpm in dogs or >220 bpm in cats
Objective:	Ensure adequate perfusion. Decrease heart rate if required

1. Check blood pressure

- Is hypovolaemia a possible cause? If so, consider fluid bolus.
- Is the heart rate affecting cardiac output? Poor pulses? Deficits?
- Hypertension + tachycardia could indicate pain, inadequate depth of anaesthesia or sympathetic storm.

2. Ensure appropriate anaesthetic depth

- Check and correct if required to stop animal moving.

3. Ensure adequate analgesia

- Opioids:
  - Fentanyl 1–5 µg/kg
  - Methadone 0.1 mg/kg
  - May need intermittent positive-pressure ventilation.
- Ketamine: 0.1–0.5 mg/kg i.v.
- Medetomidine: 0.5–1 µg/kg diluted and titrated slowly to effect over 5 mins (use half dose if dexmedetomidine).

4. Check electrocardiogram (ECG)

- If supraventricular, consider:
  - Opioids:
    - Fentanyl 1–5 µg/kg
    - Methadone 0.1 mg/kg
    - May need intermittent positive-pressure ventilation
  - Beta-blockers: esmolol 0.05–0.5 mg/kg then 25–200 µg/kg/min.
- If ventricular, consider:
  - Lidocaine (dogs): 2 mg/kg boluses (up to 3) then 50–100 µg/kg/h
  - Then magnesium 40 mg/kg followed by 15 mg/kg/h
  - Or beta-blockers: esmolol 0.05–0.5 mg/kg slow i.v. then 25–200 µg/kg/min.

Nearest location for **Lidocaine without adrenaline**

5. If no ECG is available:

- Assess pulse and heart rate
  - Is there an arrhythmia?
  - Are there pulse deficits?
  - Check for fluid responsiveness (unlikely to be hypovolaemia if the heart rate is >180 bpm in dogs or 240 bpm in cats) by administering a bolus of isotonic crystalloid over 5–10 minutes and reassess blood pressure (dogs: 10 ml/kg, cats and rabbits: 5 ml/kg)
- If no obvious arrhythmia, opioids as above
- If arrhythmia present, consider lidocaine as above after considering point (6).

6. Consider electrolyte abnormalities

- Is an electrolyte disturbance likely (K^+ or Ca^{2+} or Mg^{2+})? If yes, check and correct as required.

Causes of tachycardia
Sympathetic origin
• Baroreceptor reflex (see **Hypotension** checklist)   • Pain/nociception   • Inadequate depth of anaesthesia   • Hormonal: hyperthyroidism (thyroid storm), primary adrenergic (sympathetic storm – phaeochromocytoma)
Pharmacological
• Anticholinergics   • Beta-agonists
Primary cardiac
• Primary arrhythmia (supraventricular tachycardia, atrial fibrillation, arrhythmogenic right ventricular cardiomyopathy)   • Myocardial disease (dilated cardiomyopathy, hypertrophic cardiomyopathy mitral valve disease)   • Myocardial injury
Other
• Ventricular tachycardia due to abdominal/inflammatory disease   • Electrolyte abnormalities (e.g. hypokalaemia, Ca^{2+} abnormalities, hypomagnesaemia)

Hyperkalaemia – myocardial toxicity

Description: Increase in serum K^+ leading to myocardial toxicity and arrhythmia

Objective: Restore myocardial membrane stability and correct hyperkalaemia

1. **Stop any fluids with supplemental potassium**
   - Does not include Hartmann's solution; only fluids where additional potassium has been added.

2. **Check electrocardiogram**

3. **Stabilize myocardium**

   Where bradycardia and signs of hyperkalaemic toxicity are present, use calcium boroglucate:
   - 50 mg/kg over 5–20 minutes = 50–100 mg/kg of 10% solution i.v.
   - Diluted with saline to twice the volume
   - Can repeat 2–3 times
   - Effects will last approximately 15–20 minutes.

   Nearest location for **Calcium borogluconate**

4. **Reduce potassium levels**

   Dilution:
   - If patient is hypoperfused, administer isotonic crystalloids (lactated Ringer's solution or 0.9% NaCl) as required to restore adequate perfusion.

   Increased uptake:
   - Soluble insulin:
     - 0.5 IU/kg insulin as a bolus alongside glucose 1–1.5 g/IU insulin
     - Followed by glucose at a minimum of 1–1.5 g/IU insulin over 4–6 hours; monitor blood glucose and alter dose to effect.

Section 1

Section 2

Section 3

4. Reduce potassium levels *continued*

Increased uptake:

- Bicarbonate:
  - 0.5–1 mEq/kg over 20–30 minutes (1 ml/kg of 8.4% 1 mmol/ml bicarbonate diluted in saline) or
  - Bicarbonate deficit mmol = weight*0.2*BE (Give one-third to one-half of this and reassess).
- Beta-adrenergic agonists (can be considered although effect is mainly theoretical):
  - Salbutamol inhaler 100 µg per 'puff':
    - 1 puff for small-sized animals
    - 2 for medium-sized animals
    - 3 for large-sized animals.

5. Correct underlying cause

- Check abdomen/bladder/urine output.
- Consider massive cellular damage (e.g. trauma, neoplasia).
- Consider hypoadrenocorticism.
- Inadvertent over-administration of potassium-containing fluids.

Anaphylaxis and allergic reactions

Description:	Urticaria, vasodilation, bronchoconstriction, tachycardia
Objective:	Remove trigger. Reverse bronchospasm/vasodilation. Control immune reaction

1. **Remove trigger**
   - Stop all potential triggers (antibiotics are the most common).

2. **Ensure fraction of inspired oxygen (FiO_2) is 100%**

3. **Consider pharmacological intervention**

   If a mild reaction, administer antihistamines/corticosteroids:
   - Chlorphenamine 5–10 mg i.m.
   - Ranitidine 1.5 mg/kg i.m.
   - Consider dexamethasone 0.1–0.5 mg/kg.

   Nearest location for **Chlorphenamine**

   If severe, administer adrenergic agents:
   - Adrenaline 1–10 µg/kg q1–2min or 0.1–2 µg/kg/min after bolus
   - Chlorphenamine 5–10 mg i.m.
   - Salbutamol inhaler 100 µg per 'puff':
     - 1 puff for small-sized animals
     - 2 for medium-sized animals
     - 3 for large-sized animals.

   Nearest location for **Adrenaline**

4. **Consider terminating procedure**

5. **Write warning note on animal's file**

Pulmonary embolism

Description:	Sudden drop in end-tidal carbon dioxide ($ET'CO_2$), arrhythmia (tachy- or bradycardia), hypotension, hypoxaemia and potentially cardiopulmonary arrest caused by large blockage of pulmonary vasculature by air, thrombus, fat or other (e.g. bone cement). May be seen in spinal surgery, hip replacement, orthopaedic surgery, amputation and lower limb surgery
Objective:	Support cardiovascular and respiratory systems whilst emboli dissipate, shift emboli from right atrium/pulmonary artery through cardiopulmonary resuscitation

1. **Stop further embolization**
   - Stop procedure.
   - Stop nitrous oxide (N_2O).
   - Flood surgical site with saline or apply direct pressure.
   - If operating on limbs, tourniquet the limb above the surgery site and lower the limb below level of the heart if possible.
   - Check all intravenous lines.

2. **Start cardiopulmonary resuscitation if signs are severe**

3. **Ventilate with fraction of inspired oxygen (FiO_2) 100%**
   - Mechanically or by hand.

4. **Monitor for further deterioration**
   Paying special attention to:
   - Dropping $ET'CO_2$
   - Arrhythmia
   - Blood pressure and pulse quality
   - Oxygen saturation (SpO_2).

5. **Treat symptomatically**
   - Animal may benefit from a fluid bolus:
     - 10 ml/kg isotonic crystalloid.

Troubleshooting: pulse waveforms and pulse oximetry

Description: Commonly pulse oximeters will give erroneous readings, either inaccurate oxygen saturation (SpO_2) or pulse rates

Objective: Check validity of SpO_2 and pulse rate measurements to help ensure true adverse events are identified and treated and unnecessary treatments are not administered

> **Warning: Pulse oximeters commonly give erroneous readings; however, low SpO_2 measurements should always be assessed**

Pulse signal quality

- Are the pulses believable?
  - Do they have a good shape?
  - Are they of a good height?
- Do they correspond with manually palpated pulses and is the heart rate similar?

Normal plethysmograph trace

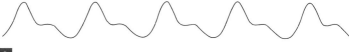

A

Hyperdynamic plethysmograph trace (vasodilation)

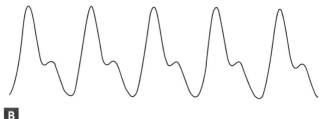

B

Weak plethysmograph trace (hypovolaemia, vasoconstriction, low cardiac output)

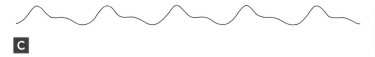

C

Signal interference (e.g. ambient light)

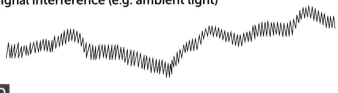

D

- Signals (A) and (B) are likely to be accurate and can therefore be believed and acted on if necessary.
- Signal (C) may well be erroneous due to poor perfusion. Attempt to improve signal quality and check other parameters for warning signs of crisis.
- Anything with a lower signal quality than Signal (C) should be considered with caution as error is likely. Attempts should be made to improve signal quality. Check other parameters to ensure the animal is stable.
- Signal (D) will be erroneous – there is interference and not obvious pulses. Attempts should be made to improve signal quality.

Methods to improve signal quality

- Move the probe to a different site.
- Use a wet swab between the probe and the animal.
- Protect the probe from ambient light.
- Ensure adequate perfusion (correct blood pressure issues).
- Avoid using vasoconstricting drugs.

Troubleshooting: capnography

34

Description:	The capnograph trace can be affected by several factors and therefore measurements may not be representative
Objective:	Check validity of capnography traces and end-tidal carbon dioxide ($ET'CO_2$) and respiratory rate measurements to help ensure true adverse events are identified and treated and that unnecessary treatments are not administered in false adverse events

> **Warning: Capnographs will rarely give $ET'CO_2$ measurements higher than they really are. If the $ET'CO_2$ is above 65 mmHg, start mechanical or manual ventilation and address underlying cause**

Normal trace

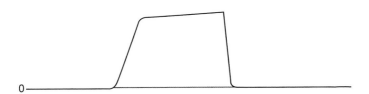

0

No capnograph trace

Flat line at zero.

Causes	Intervention
Capnograph not connected	Check capnograph is attached to breathing system
Airway not patent	Perform **Rapid situational assessment.** Ensure airway patent via administration of a manual breath. Visually check airway. Change endotracheal tube, unkink or suction as required

No capnograph trace *continued*

Causes	Intervention
Apnoea or respiratory arrest or no cardiac output	Perform **Rapid situational assessment**. Start cardiopulmonary resuscitation or intermittent positive-pressure ventilation as necessary or perform **Post-induction apnoea** checklist
Airway disconnection	Perform **Rapid situational assessment**. Hand ventilation should reveal a leak. Reconnect and administer another breath if the animal is not breathing. Follow the **post-induction apnoea** checklist
Capnograph zeroing or calibrating – capnograph just turned on or routine electronic main-tenance during use	Perform **Rapid situational assessment**. Rule out apnoea, disconnection and airway failure; check animal is breathing, ventilate as required to maintain oxygen saturation (SpO_2) >93–95%, check monitor for signs of zeroing or calibration, wait until capnograph warmed up

Lower than expected ET'CO$_2$

Normal trace but lower than expected for animal's breathing (e.g. respiratory rate and apparent tidal volume).

Causes	Intervention
Poor cardiac output – reduced CO_2 delivery to lungs	Perform **Rapid situational assessment**, rule out cardiopulmonary arrest and hypotension. Start relevant checklists
Poor tidal volume – animal not taking deep breaths so ET'CO$_2$ not representative	Perform **Rapid situational assessment**, rule out cardiopulmonary arrest and hypotension. When administering hand-ventilated breath, assess if ET'CO$_2$ increases, consider mechanical ventilation if it does
High fresh gas flow to tidal volume ratio; with non-rebreathing systems the high fresh gas flow may dilute small tidal volumes and reduce ET'CO$_2$	Perform **Rapid situational assessment**, rule out cardiopulmonary arrest and hypotension. Reduce fresh gas flow and see if ET'CO$_2$ increases, be aware ET'CO$_2$ may be measured lower than it really is, consider mainstream capnography if available
Capnograph not calibrated to anaesthetic gases being used	Check capnograph is not calibrated to a gas mixture containing nitrous oxide (N_2O)

Troubleshooting: capnography *continued*

Higher than expected CO_2

Normal trace but higher than expected for animal's breathing (e.g. respiratory rate and apparent tidal volume).

Causes	Intervention
Hypoventilation	Start mechanical or hand ventilation. If depth of anaesthesia 'too deep' then can try to lower vaporizer setting. Will need short-term ventilation
If N_2O being used: • N_2O administration will falsely elevate $ET'CO_2$ unless corrections are made by the capnograph	Recalibrate capnograph (turn off and back on again, sampling the gas mixture being used) or set gas mixture on capnograph set-up

Failure of capnograph to return to zero baseline

Rebreathing.

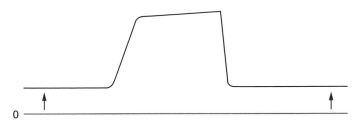

Causes	Intervention
Non-rebreathing systems: inadequate fresh gas flow	Increase fresh gas flow
Rebreathing systems: soda lime exhausted	Check soda lime and change circle system if necessary, increasing fresh gas flow may improve
Rebreathing systems: one-way valves stuck	Check valves, change canister if valves not working
Increased dead space (probably will not respond to increasing fresh gas flow)	Check endotracheal tube and shorten if needed, remove unnecessary connectors, consider ventilating
Short shallow respirations/ panting	Check depth – increase vaporizer and ventilate until under control, consider administering additional analgesia

Shark fin appearance during expiratory upstroke

Bronchoconstriction or airway obstruction.

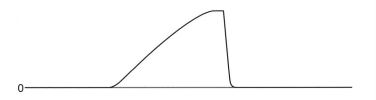

Causes	Intervention
Anaphylaxis	Check skin and face for urticaria, check blood pressure and heart rate; see **Anaphylaxis and allergic reactions** checklist
Bronchospasm	Airway obstruction with no cutaneous signs; follow **Bronchoconstriction** checklist

Normal trace but large rapid drop in ET'CO$_2$

Rapid decline in ET'CO$_2$ over a short number of breaths, most common during ventilation or with a sudden drop in ET'CO$_2$.

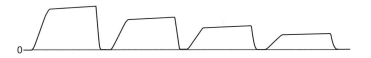

Causes	Intervention
Impending cardiopulmonary arrest – sudden decrease in cardiac output reduces blood flow and CO$_2$ delivery to the lungs	Perform **Rapid situational assessment** and consider cardiopulmonary resuscitation or follow **Hypotension** checklist
Embolism – air, thrombus or other material (e.g. bone cement) lodges in pulmonary vasculature causing sudden increase in alveolar dead space leading to areas of poorly perfused lung	Perform **Rapid situational assessment** and follow **Pulmonary embolism** checklist

Troubleshooting: capnography *continued*

Rounded trace with drop in ET'CO$_2$

Declining ET'CO$_2$ levels with capnograph showing blunted corners.

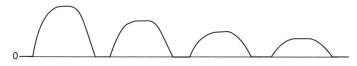

Causes	Intervention
Leak around endotracheal tube reduces CO$_2$ able to be measured by capnograph	Perform **Rapid situational assessment**, rule out cardiopulmonary arrest, hand ventilation should reveal leak, inflate cuff as required

Slow gradual drop-off of CO$_2$

Trace forms a 'tail' during the inspiratory phase.

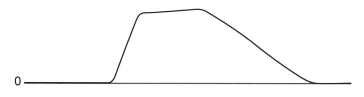

Causes	Intervention
Prolonged expiratory pause – where stroke volume is high with a prolonged expiratory pause, large volume blood flow through pulmonary vessels causes additional CO$_2$ to be expelled during every heartbeat	If ET'CO$_2$ is high, start mechanical ventilation, check depth and adjust if required – may not need to do anything if ET'CO$_2$ is normal

Cardiogenic oscillations

Jagged tail and drop-off of CO$_2$ during the inspiratory phase.

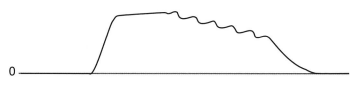

Causes	Intervention
Where there is a prolonged expiratory pause and the animal does not breath, in following expiration, the CO$_2$ is slowly reduced by the fresh gas flow diluting it	If ET'CO$_2$ is high, start mechanical ventilation, check depth and adjust if required; may not need to do anything if ET'CO$_2$ is normal

Notes:

Index of checklists

Section 1

Section 2

Section 3